America's Healthcare Plan
A Strategy for Achieving Quality Care

A Facebook Book

Scott Hallal-Negishi

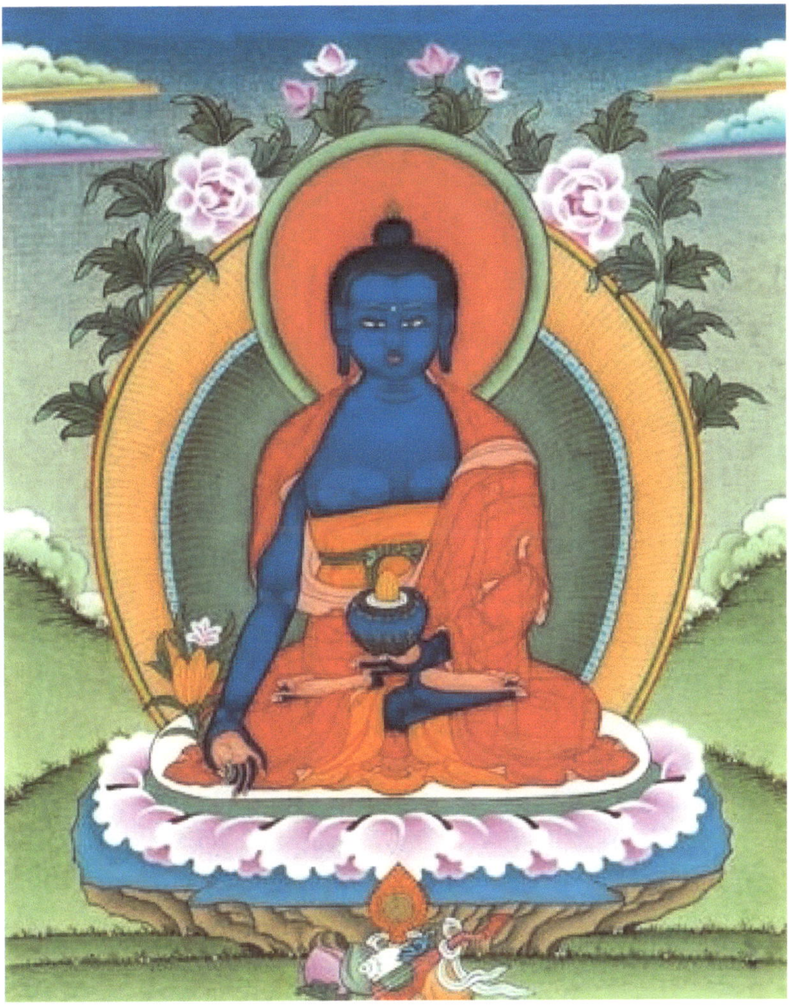

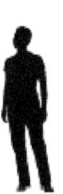

Kinutaro Publishing

ISBN-13: 978-1522870470

ISBN-10: 1522870474

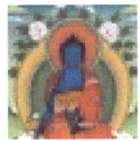

America's Healthcare Plan: A Strategy for Achieving Quality Care

About

America's healthcare system is progressing towards quality care. What solutions will help in successfully implementing this new type of medical care?

Description

America's healthcare system is progressing towards quality care. Physicians are to be paid based on the outcome of their treatment methods and provided incentives so that patients do not return for further care. The payment for quality care does not correlate with the current payment system based on services provided. Hospitals and other organizations are attempting to offer quality care services to their patients, and these organizations are setting the example for this type of care. The current healthcare system is financially strained and hospitals and small physician practices take great steps assuring they continue to offer the best care to their patients. Under a quality-based healthcare system, the survival of hospitals and small physician practices will be even more difficult and the incentives to recruit and pay the best doctors will also be more challenging because quality-care services are designed to decrease cost. There is a solution however. The American concept of quality-care decreases cost, but it also decreases incentive; however, the Tibetan concept of quality-care decreases cost, but it rather increases incentive because Tibetan medicine is designed as a quality-care system. Through a Tibetan-based healthcare system, quality-care services can be provided that decrease unnecessary procedures, which cut back time, and increase payments on services offered.

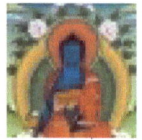

[America's Healthcare Plan: A Strategy for Achieving Quality Care](#)

[July 16](#) via [mobile](#)

My strategy, plan, and quality-care method are now complete.

[1Like](#) · · [Share](#)

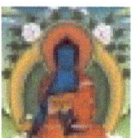

[America's Healthcare Plan: A Strategy for Achieving Quality Care](#)

[July 15](#)

What is important to the population?

[Like](#) · · [Share](#)

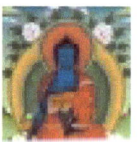

[America's Healthcare Plan: A Strategy for Achieving Quality Care](#)

[July 15](#)

Seniority in Minnesota is reflected through the community and by community I mean both relationships and neighborhood/city.

[Like](#) · · [Share](#)

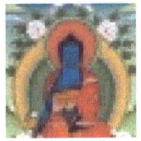

[America's Healthcare Plan: A Strategy for Achieving Quality Care](#)

[July 15](#)

Moving on to Minnesota. A completely different picture of America, where the Arctic Air swoops down untouched to the open plains.

[2Like](#) · · [Share](#)

[America's Healthcare Plan: A Strategy for Achieving Quality Care](#)

Similar to Hawaii, in Minnesota the deep roots of community are attained over time.

[July 15 at 5:16pm](#) · [Like](#)

[America's Healthcare Plan: A Strategy for Achieving Quality Care](#)

This could be a global concept, but I am not sure.

[July 15 at 5:17pm](#) · [Like](#)

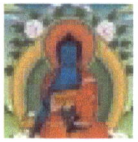

[America's Healthcare Plan: A Strategy for Achieving Quality Care](#)

[July 15](#)

I have decided to make seniority the basis of my healthcare strategy. This was based on my analysis of Hawaii, which, in a 'vacuum' environment, or utopia, the longer someone has lived in Hawaii, the better housing they are entitled to.

[Like](#) · · [Share](#)

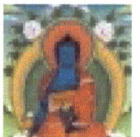

[America's Healthcare Plan: A Strategy for Achieving Quality Care](#)

[July 15](#)

I was messaging my friend in regards to some work that was completed on population health and physician networks, and I mentioned to him the following, which emphasizes the need for a revised, high-quality payment system for America's healthcare:

"Well there is a lot of money in the topic I am investigating; America's healthcare system. I realized this after getting more into this topic and researching what grants were available. I found that Medicare, Medicaid, and CHIP need to be revised for a payment system for quality-care. The grant is for organizations, so I do not qualify, but to give you a sense of the need, the floor for the grant is $1,000,000 and the ceiling is $30,000,000, and this grant is geared more for the concept of the system, so no real technology is necessary or required."

[1Like](#) · · [Share](#)

America's Healthcare Plan: A Strategy for Achieving Quality Care

The nature of my interest in the grant was that I was thinking grant money could be used to conduct a survey of America in the same manner that Gandhi traveled across India gaining a clear picture of the politics and challenges facing the people.

July 15 at 12:36am · Like

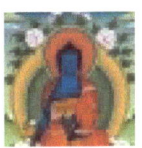

America's Healthcare Plan: A Strategy for Achieving Quality Care

July 15

Tibetan history associates housing with status in most contexts. Status refers to class and title/job. My discussion will analyze housing in a similar context.

Like · · Share

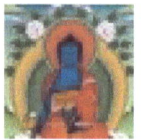

[America's Healthcare Plan: A Strategy for Achieving Quality Care](#)

July 14

The amount of time you have been in Hawaii is very important and it has a direct and indirect relationship with housing. When I say the amount of time, I am referring to the family background, in which an individual's family could have immigrated to Hawaii perhaps four generations in the past, and the other context is that someone recently moved to Hawaii, and they are the first generation.

Like · · Share

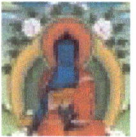

[America's Healthcare Plan: A Strategy for Achieving Quality Care](#)

July 14

Although there exists a sense of equality similar to the American Dream, the Dream of Hawaii is quite different than that of the continental US or mainland. There are many similarities, which I will refer to, but across the islands of Hawaii, there is an overwhelming sense of what it means to be Hawaiian still rooted in the ideology of people from Hawaii and people who come to live in Hawaii.

Like · · Share

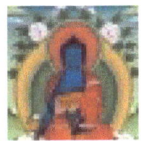

[America's Healthcare Plan: A Strategy for Achieving Quality Care](#)

[July 14](#)

I spent seven years in Hawaii having graduated from the University of Hawaii and worked in the healthcare industry for a period of time after that. One of the most important aspects of society that I became exposed to during my time in Hawaii was the integration of people of different social and cultural backgrounds in day-to-day living.

This concept of equality reflects the American Dream in that all people are entitled to pursue financial success and all people are equal when it comes to their pursuits. There are direct correlations between this concept of equality and housing.

[1Like](#) · · [Share](#)

[America's Healthcare Plan: A Strategy for Achieving Quality Care](#)

I think this social concept of equality in Hawaii is rooted in the Hawaiian ethic that all people and all living beings are welcome in Hawaii.

[July 14 at 9:27pm](#) · [Like](#)

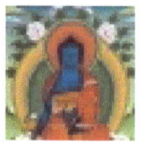

America's Healthcare Plan: A Strategy for Achieving Quality Care

July 14

Like Keaomelemele, Hawaiian stories start in one place, then move in both time and place to recount something important and valuable, and maybe return to the story at hand way down the way, but like time itself, the story may take place in the most applicable of contexts without a clear distinction, left in the eye of the beholder.

This is why I am now including a paper I wrote called "Housing and Health: Success Through Data Coordination"

Two important processes that characterize the assessment function of public health are to monitor health status to identify community health problems and to diagnose and investigate health problems and health hazards in the community. Housing and health care are both in a state of crisis, particularly for families with limited means. Assessing housing and health through a scientific examination of the efficacy of healthy housing interventions can help to improve both health and housing, reducing the cost of health care services. Specifically, an assessment can provide a clearer understanding of the demographic and socioeconomic determinants of health, community assets, environmental and behavioral risks, and quality of life. Individual participation in a community's assessment can play an important role in community health, which will balance overreliance on data and expert opinion and provide new insights into factors affecting community health. Studies in housing and health have historically been fragmented because there is a lack of organization in studies, determinants, and outcomes. Shifts in the utilization of qualitative data and quantitative data have added to the lack of clear understanding of the results that a variety and multitude of studies have produced. This paper attempts to assess the results on housing and health by describing results from different studies and research, and it provides a recommendation for improvements in housing through actions at the community level. The greatest gains that I can hope for by assessing studies on housing and health are to increase the amount of coordination between individuals and entities that contribute to these issues at all levels and to encourage more assessments to be conducted that will further organize the research that has been conducted on housing and health in order to improve quality of life for everyone. Health is a fundamental resource to the individual, the community, and to society. When people are healthy, they are better able to work, learn, build a good life, and contribute to society. That being said, reaching a healthy population requires better living conditions, better quality of life, and less stress. By first improving living conditions, which will reduce stress and improve the quality of life, people will have better health, and, like a cycle, better health will feed into the community and society, thus improving living conditions and quality of life. Older cities in America have declined in quality due to the economic shifts that have marked the last two decades. One example showing this is that employment opportunities have been removed from low-income neighborhoods. Businesses do not want to build offices, plants, or stores in these areas. New approaches to rebuild low-income communities are a vital necessity. One approach is the Capacity-Focused Alternative method. Rather than implementing programs addressing poor living conditions, this approach is to develop policies and activities based on the composition of a neighborhood. For example, what the capacities, skills, and assets are for low-income people. The reasoning behind the Capacity-Focused Alternative method is that historic evidence indicates that significant community development only takes place when local community people are committed to investing themselves and their resources in the effort. By identifying capacities and assets of both individual and organizational, the process of community regeneration can begin. Once identified, the regenerating community can begin to assemble its assets and capacities into new combinations, new structures of opportunity, new sources of income and control, and new possibilities for production. One important focus is to restructure financial resource streams which originate outside the neighborhood. These are funds that are controlled by institutions outside the neighborhood but used for community-building purposes like state and federal funding distributed through programs. As mentioned, programs are to be replaced by policies and activities based on the capacities, skills, and assets of a neighborhood. One approach of this type is to develop tools and models for converting public expenditures into local development investments.

A report was recently published by the National Low Income Housing Coalition titled "Dark Before the Storm: A Picture of Low Income Renters' Housing Needs before the Great Recession from the 2005-2007 American Community Survey," that provides further definition of the housing problem. This report exhibits results of an analysis of new U.S. Department of Housing and Urban Development (HUD) data that use the 2005-2007 American Community Survey (ACS) to replicate indicators of housing need last released using Census 2000 data. Over three-fourths of low income renter households in the U.S. were said to have had a least one housing problem in 2005-2007. Low income households are at a disadvantage in the housing market due to the severe cost burden they face, which is to say that 63% paid more than half of their income on rent and utilities. This population cannot afford quality living conditions without sacrificing their health. When low-income families pay more than half of their income on rent, they spend 30% less on food and 70% less on health care. In 2000, 70% of the 8,100,000 low income renter households lived in unaffordable housing. This population grew over the next five to seven years. By 2005-2007, 76% of the 9,200,000 low income renter households had unaffordable housing costs. Income limits used in this data are defined by HUD and take into account HUD adjustments in determining the 30%, 50% and 80% threshold of area median income and geography. These adjustments provide a more detailed analysis over the standard Census and ACS. Policy makers, researchers, and local governments use the adjusted data to better understand household needs. The National Housing Trust Fund (NHTF) is one example of a program that utilizes adjusted data, also referred to as Comprehensive Housing Affordability Strategy data. NHTF creates and preserves affordable housing for renters exhibiting the greatest need.

Data collection methods are constantly being updated, revised, and improved to better reflect the population and to capture the housing needs in a changing environment. The ACS reaches nationwide to approximately three million households each year. Areas the ACS covers include social, economic, demographic and housing. The ACS is a shorter form as compared to the Census, and in 2010 the ACS replaced the Census "long form" and allowed more frequent data collection. The survey is conducted in one-year, three-year and five-year data sets. One-year data sets document changes over time while three-year and five-year data sets provide an aggregate of data of the time period. In analyzing the ACS data, it was discovered that the one-year data sets revealed a year-to-year growth in monthly rents from 2007 to 2010 that exceeded income gains. Rents are rising faster than income, as the data showed. Wary of this trend, Americans are choosing in greater numbers to rent rather than buy. The demand for rental units is therefore on the rise, causing a decrease in affordable housing, which is increasing competition for units that remain available on the market. When a homeowner is forced to sell in the event of a foreclosure, a loss of a job, or other financial hardship, the loss can be traumatic, and especially devastating for Latino families according to a study by The National Council of La Raza (NCLR). A house is two-thirds of a Latino family's household wealth. Losing their home therefore puts their assets and entire financial future at risk. NCLR conducted 25 interviews with Latino families and it was determined that foreclosures placed a heavy burden on the entire family affecting their mental and emotional health as well as their relationships. With money even tighter, some families reported skipping trips to the doctor or cutting back on medications to save money. Both parents and children exhibited signs of anxiety, depression, stress, and tension. Parents expressed concern about their children's health. This is understandable because without a savings, families could not afford quality healthcare or medical care in the event of an emergency. Access to quality healthcare has become a social indicator of "quality of life" in the United States. The Bureau of Health Services Research has developed a need-based empirical indicator of the access concept, which is the use/disability ratio, or the number of physician visits per 100 days of disability experienced. Utilization of services by the population at risk is shown to be relative to their expressed need for care. If improvements are to be made in "quality of life," access to healthcare must be improved, and in order to improve access, the housing infrastructure has to also be improved.

Subsidized housing buffers families from food insecurity and other health risks according to research by Children's HealthWatch. A housing subsidy limits the percent of income paid in rent, which frees up resources for other household necessities, including food. Children's HealthWatch found that children living in subsidized housing were more likely to be food secure and less likely to be seriously underweight than children whose families were on the wait list for subsidized housing. Poor children without subsidies have higher rates of iron deficiency, malnutrition, and stunting of growth.

Poor housing conditions are a concern for subsidized housing as well as non-subsidized housing because of the high demand for rental units, which causes the quality of affordable housing to diminish. Congress established the Healthy Homes Initiative (HHI) to develop and implement a program of research and demonstration projects that would address multiple housing-related problems affecting the health of children. HHI strives to identify multiple housing deficiencies that affect health, safety, and quality of life and to take actions to reduce or eliminate the health risks related to poor quality housing with interventions in four areas: excess moisture; dust; ventilation and control of toxins; and tenant education in high-risk housing areas. The Robert Wood Johnson Foundation Commission to Build a Healthier America's recent report focused on three aspects of residential housing and their links to health including the physical conditions within homes; conditions in the neighborhoods surrounding homes; and housing affordability. From a medical standpoint, lead poisoning irreversibly affects brain and nervous system development, resulting in lower intelligence and reading disabilities. The Robert Wood Johnson Foundation Commission to Build a Healthier America reported that an estimated 310,000 children ages one to five have elevated blood lead levels. Housing conditions such as water leaks, poor ventilation, dirty carpets, and pest infestation can lead to an increase in mold, mites, and other allergens that are known to be associated with poor health. Indoor allergens and damp housing conditions can develop into respiratory conditions including asthma, which is the most common chronic disease among children. Healthcare data shows that forty percent of diagnosed asthma among children are believed to be attributable to residential exposures.

Other health concerns from housing include lung cancer and respiratory illness from radon, tobacco smoke, pollutants from heating and cooking with gas, volatile organic compounds, and asbestos.

Housing conditions are vitally important to health. Conditions in neighborhoods and communities have an equal impact on health. The shortage of affordable housing limits family's choices about where they can live. Typically, low income families migrate to substandard housing in unsafe, overcrowded neighborhoods with higher rates of poverty and fewer community assets like parks, education, jobs, and recreation facilities. Socioeconomic characteristics of neighborhoods have shown to affect short-term and long-term health quality and longevity. Socioeconomic characteristics are typically associated with crime, violence, and pollution, which need to be controlled in addition to building community assets and infrastructure. Relationships can greatly influence psychological health, because having trust in fellow residents means an ease of mind. Not only is access to healthcare important, a strong and healthy community needs access to grocery stores and good food in order to eat right. Neighborhoods are diverse, even within small cities or towns. Neighborhoods differ in economic and social resources and their income-status can be a health determiner. Housing discrimination prohibits some low-income families from living in healthy communities. Racial and ethnic discrimination usually become associated with certain neighborhoods depending on income level, and this further compounds the disadvantage of a community.

The greatest gains, according to Turnock in Public Health: What It Is and How It Works, will come from what people do or do not do for themselves, individually and collectively. Communities need to conduct assessments of themselves and determine what assets they possess. Needs or problems will always be evident; however, a shift in perspective needs to be made in order to make improvements because the current needs approach is not making progress. This is because assessing a community by their needs or problems will lead to policy interventions that are based on needs or problems. When assessments are made based on their assets, socioeconomic factors are brought into the model that will address a community's capacities, skills and assets. Socioeconomic factors represent both the infrastructure of a community and the active lives of people that change on a daily basis. Turnock states that community health improvement seldom occurs from the actions of outside interests alone, and that the most successful community development efforts are driven by the commitment of those investing themselves and their resources in the effort. Rather than turning to state and federal funding, communities need to build a better economic foundation that contributes to their overall economic and social success. These building blocks will help address the needs and problems. In addition to addressing community needs and problems, individual households will see change because of their own contributions to the community's success.

Improvements in the economic foundation mean their own economic foundation will be improved. This might mean better jobs, more access to education, better grocery stores, and less stress. Bringing together people and organizations through citizen associations, cultural organizations, communications organizations, and religious organizations can lead to greater unity and a better possibility to contribute at a community level. Individual organizations do not always lead to effective results due to the heterogeneity of a community, ratio to the entire population, and the complex rules and system of the government. Two older projects called Turning Point and Community Voices constructed a road map for communities and their partners in which "health improvement and other positive outcomes resulted from collaborations that were sustained over the long term, that institutionalize effective programs and processes, and that mobilize and utilize all available resources to deal with evolving challenges and population health issues." Coordinating results from studies, programs and reports will help contribute to the collaborations that need to take place at the community level in order to see improvements in health. The studies in this paper were not necessarily connected, but they help shine light on a single topic of housing and health. This type of work to bring different studies together to further a topic is not new. The majority of scientific and professional papers require various sources to clarify the central idea of their report. However, the results of connecting studies as a means to improve care through coordination have not been fully realized. More focus should be made in the coordination of studies, programs, and data. Information technology has made this possible, so now it should be utilized. This needs to be realized quickly too before the management of data becomes too convoluted to process and identify simple connections that can lead to improvements in health and socioeconomic factors to better off communities.

References
Turnock BJ. Public Health: What It Is and How It Works. Sudbury, Massachusetts: Jones and Bartlett Publishers' 2009.
National Center for Healthy Housing. Housing Interventions and Health: A Review of the Evidence. 2009.
Institute of Medicine of the National Academies. The Future of the Public's Health in the 21st Century. Washington, D.C.: The National Academies Press; 2003.
McKnight JL, Kretzmann J. Mapping community capacity. Evanston, IL: Center for Urban Affairs and Policy Research, Northwestern University; 1990.
DeCrappeo M, Pelletiere D. Dark Before the Storm: A Picture of Low Income Renters' Housing Needs before the Great Recession from the 2005-2007 American Community Survey. National Low Income Housing Coalition. 2011.
Conroy, K. Housing and Health: Making a Stronger Case for Affordable

Housing. MLP Boston; 2009.

National Low Income Housing Coalition. Housing Spotlight: Renters' Growing Pain. Volume 1, Issue 1. 2011.

Bowdler J, Quercia R, Smith D A. The Foreclosure Generation: The Long-Term Impact of the Housing Crisis on Latino Children and Families. The National Council of La Raza. 2010.

Aday LA, Andersen R. A Framework for the Study of Access to Medical Care. Health Serv Res. 1974; Fall: 208-220.

Children's Healthwatch, Medical-Legal Partnership. Rx for Hunger: Affordable Housing. 2009.

Robert Wood Johnson Foundation Commission to Build a Healthier America. Where We Live Matters for Out Health: The Links Between Housing and Health. Issue Brief 2: Housing and Health. 2008.

Like · · Share

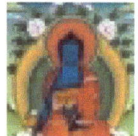

America's Healthcare Plan: A Strategy for Achieving Quality Care

July 14

Here is info and a diagram of my socioeconomic initiative on debt injections:

Socioeconomic Model for a Public Health Solution to Improving Health

Dollar injections when encountering debt
Reaching for Top of the Mountain
Eliminating limitations of dollar
Attempting to make the dollar infinite
Wealth is determined by how much one gives rather than how much one accumulates.
Dollar will boost immunity because of less stress.

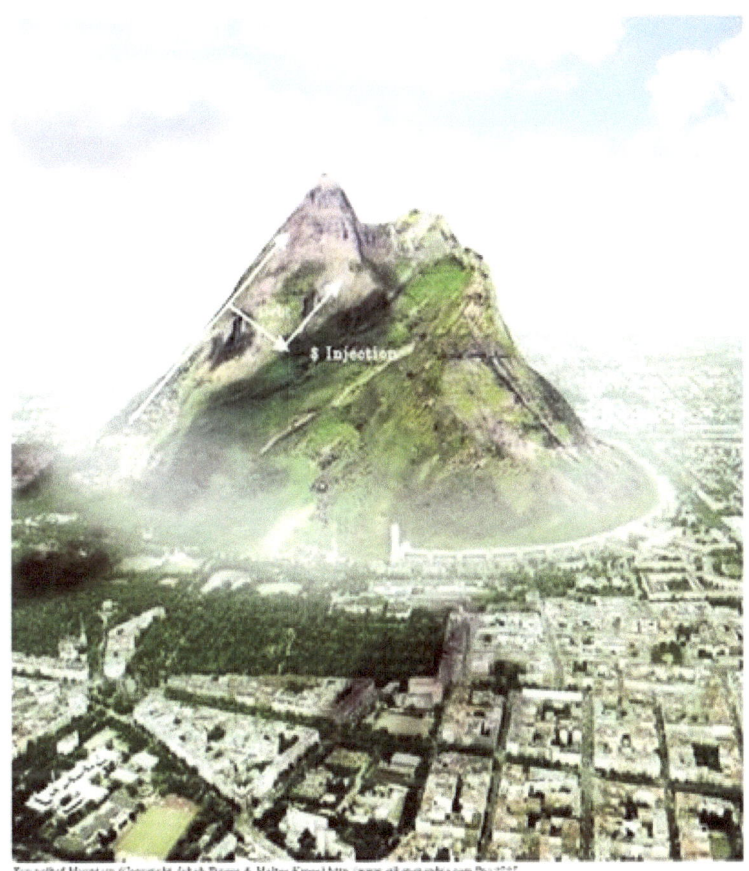

Tempelhof Mountain (Copyright Jakob Tigges & Maltes Krone) http://www.rikongraphos.com/?p=2727

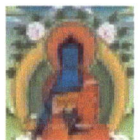

[America's Healthcare Plan: A Strategy for Achieving Quality Care](#)

[July 14](#)

As my first contributor of culture in a system of culture, I will focus on housing. Housing is a very large part of the organization and structure of Tibetan history, and I feel it provides a good representation of the people.

[1Like](#) · · [Share](#)

[America's Healthcare Plan: A Strategy for Achieving Quality Care](#)

The first place I will begin my discuss on housing is Hawaii.

[July 14 at 12:33am](#) · [Like](#)

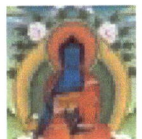

You Were Born for a Reason is best read together with the Buddhist parable "The Reality of Mankind," brought to attention of Leo Tolstoy stated as follows:

Buddhism is the teachings of the Buddha, also known as Sakyamuni Buddha. He is called this way because he was from the Sakya clan in India.
When learning Buddhism, the most important thing to know is the purpose of listening to its teachings. Sakyamuni explained the objective of listening to Buddhism in a famous parable.
This parable shocked Leo Tolstoy, renowned Russian writer of War and Peace. Tolstoy said, "I have never heard any parables which reveal human reality as genuine as this Eastern fable."
During the time of Sakyamuni, a king by the name of Shoko, decided to attend a lecture of Buddhism. Sakyamuni was pleased at his attendance since it tended to be difficult for persons in power to hear Buddhism due to their vanity and high position. For this reason, Sakyamuni preached about the purpose of listening to Buddhism in a parable called:
"The Reality of Mankind"
Billions of years ago, a traveler was trudging all alone across a vast wilderness. It was a lonely evening in the fall, and the cold wintry wind swept across the bitter plain. The traveler was hastening his pace toward home when suddenly, he spotted some white objects scattered along the roadside. He picked one up, wondering what it could be and to his horror discovered it was a human bone.
"Now why would there be human bones scattered around here?" the traveler wondered as he felt an eerie feeling come over him.
He cast his eyes around but saw neither a crematory nor a graveyard in the vicinity. Seized with a very chilling feeling, the traveler couldn't even take a single step forward.
As he kept staring at the white bones, he heard a weird growl and the sound of ominous footsteps coming toward him.
"What is that sound?" the traveler wondered as he looked ahead. To his terror, it was a huge tiger, fierce from starvation and charging straight for him.
Instantaneously, he realized the meaning of those bones. Travelers who had

passed here like himself had become the tiger's prey, and these bones were the remains of their dead bodies.

As soon as he realized this, he panicked even more before running back down the road he had come from with all his might. However, no matter how desperately or quickly he could run, it was still just a competition between a tiger and a human being. There was just no way he could outrun a tiger. The distance between them drew closer and closer. He could even hear the tiger's violent snort just behind him.

Somewhere in his haste, the traveler made a wrong turn leading to the edge of a steep cliff.

"Oh no!" he cried. "I've taken the wrong road!" But it was much too late to turn back now.

A pine tree stood on the top of the cliff. It was useless to climb it for safety, however, because tigers are expert tree climbers.

The traveler while running in circles around the tree – not knowing what else to do – managed to find a lifesaver. It was a wisteria vine hanging from the base of the pine tree leading down the precipice.

"Great! This'll do it!" The traveler quickly clung to the vine and narrowly escaped the hungry tiger.

The tiger, losing its prey, growled fiercely from atop the cliff.

"Thanks to this vine, I'm safe for now."

Thinking he was out of danger, the traveler casually looked down to see what it was like below him and gasped in surprise and terror.

What he saw was a vast, fathomless sea with swift currents swirling dangerously. But not just that. Amidst the whirlpool were three dragons – blue, red, and black – waiting for him to fall. Their mouths were wide open ready to devour him.

Seeing this dreadful scene below the traveler tightened his grip.

Out of luck yet again, he was now in a more desperate situation.

After hanging around for a while however, he began to feel hungry and looked around for something edible.

Suddenly upon peering upward, he discovered what horrified him the most. It was more frightening than either the menacing tiger or the three deadly dragons below him. He involuntarily cried out from the sheer terror.

Two mice, one white and the other black, had appeared from nowhere, and were taking turns gnawing the vine, his only lifeline. The traveler's face turned pale and his body was shaking in fear. He shook the vine rigorously to shoo the mice away, but to no avail. The mice just kept taking turns chewing on his wisteria vine.

But a strange phenomenon started occurring as he shook the vine. With each shake, something had come dripping down.

The traveler caught some of it with his hand and to his utter astonishment discovered it was a delicious-looking drop of honey. Instinctively, he licked it and found it to be the most delicious honey that he had ever tasted in his life. He wondered, "Why would honey be dripping down from above?" And as he looked up again he saw a beehive on the branch from which the vine hung. Hoping to taste it once more, he shook the vine again and as he hoped, more honey came dripping down.

"Once more. Just once more."

The traveler kept on licking the honey intoxicated with delight, and forgetting all the dangers he was in from the tiger, the three dragons, and even the dreadful black and white mice. All he had in mind now was how to obtain more honey. When Sakyamuni Buddha's sermon reached this point, someone in the audience shouted.

"Noble Sakya! Please stop!" It was King Shoko. "I am too frightened to hear this story anymore. How can this traveler be so foolish? How could he ever forget he was in such danger, simply being distracted by honey drops?"

"Please listen carefully, King," Sakyamuni Buddha replied. "This traveler refers to you. He represents not only you but the whole human race."

At these words, all the audience stood up in shock. Sakyamuni went on to describe how this traveler represented the reality all human beings are in now.

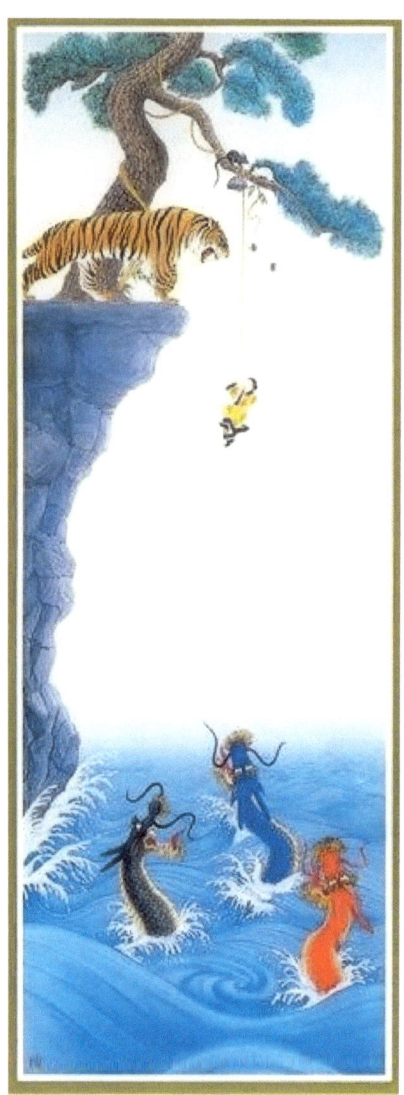

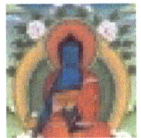

America's Healthcare Plan: A Strategy for Achieving Quality Care

July 14

This raises a good point about happiness and money introduced in the book You Were Born For a Reason: The Real Purpose of Life, which discusses that as "human beings, we have on thing in common: we search all our lives for lasting happiness, and that happiness can indeed be found. But it is not found in the places we ordinarily look, such as status, achievements, or family." Having been written by a Buddhist author and written with a Buddhist perspective, this seems applicable to a Tibetan strategy, having deep roots in Buddhism.

Like · · Share

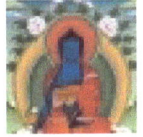

America's Healthcare Plan: A Strategy for Achieving Quality Care

July 14

Having introduced two concepts culturally related, it almost seems pertinent that happiness has a direct correlation with money. I hate to introduce this concept due to the highly controversial interpretation of money and society, but in this day and age, it might hold the most truth. I must be careful with this concept, but I might start organizing a system of culture revolving around the happiness of money in society.

Like · · Share

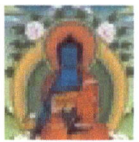

America's Healthcare Plan: A Strategy for Achieving Quality Care

July 14

The other way to interpret a system of culture is through my concept on debt injections, or simply injections. This is a public health initiative, in which money is given to people, or injected into society, for debt relief, or to boost people's finance. The point is that health is directly affected by stress, and financial problems are a huge contributor to stress. By injected people with money, enormous quantities of stress can be relieved, improving moral and improving health. There were two main drivers to this concept: one being that people are being restricted by finance and unable to pursue their ambitions, dreams, or basic life, so by injecting finances into their life, the concept of money can be dissolved and their true selves could take over, which would improve health. Two is that injections would be most beneficial if they were given to people through close encounters or through everyday relationships. This is apposed to injecting money through governmental stipends and grants, etcs. where most people are left out, especially the middle and upper classes, where financial boosts might be the most beneficial.

Like · · Share

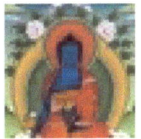

America's Healthcare Plan: A Strategy for Achieving Quality Care

July 13

I am still having troubles articulating culture through a system. I would like to think of it as the relationships between people and how they function in which case I would introduce my invention of the i, taken after the meme. I created a company called infinitorum selling i. Economic exchange happens around us everyday. infinitorum supplies the world with i, the unit of energy generated from the interaction of economic exchange.

Like · · Share

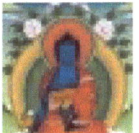

America's Healthcare Plan: A Strategy for Achieving Quality Care

July 13

Perhaps to understand and perceive culture, I must work backwards from happiness. Culture is what makes people happy, so I will focus on what makes people happy.

2Like · · Share

[Ted Schmidt](#)

Reverse engineering is a useful concept.

[July 13 at 3:15pm](#) via [mobile](#) · [Like](#)

[America's Healthcare Plan: A Strategy for Achieving Quality Care](#)

I believe it worked in my case.

[July 14 at 12:36am](#) · [Like](#) · [1](#)

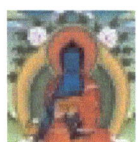

[America's Healthcare Plan: A Strategy for Achieving Quality Care](#)

[July 13](#)

Culture is more difficult than I expected to articulate. Yet vitally important in laying out the complex and intricate structure of a high-quality healthcare system. Rather than take the easy way out and further define the design of a cultural approach to system design, I will continue trying.

[Like](#) · · [Share](#)

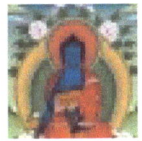

Finding the Cure for Cancer
Utilizing the Indigenous Research Method

By Scott Hallal-Negishi

My theory when entering business was that Indigenous peoples knew the most because they have been around the longest, since the time when animals and humans spoke the same language, and therefore they know the most about money, so I should learn about money from them.

My theory worked because I reached my financial goals before the age of 30, so I only thought it best that when entering the age of data, research, and analysis (Information Age) that Indigenous peoples would also know the most. My theory was right again because the Indigenous research methodology led me to what I consider the cure for cancer and my life's work: controlling air and water pollution.

Rather than explain the Indigenous research method, I will present it in this paper in the form of a first-person narrative as replicated from the book Research is Ceremony: Indigenous Research Methods, by Shawn Wilson. This narrative will support my master's paper on a cancer prevention program.

My story begins in Honolulu, Hawai'i, driving with my wife down some tropical road, talking story about my interest in Hawaiian culture and peoples, especially chanting. Chanting for me reflected my deep connection with music and my newly developed interest in Buddhism, this having been my first experience living in an area inhabited by peoples from Polynesia, Japan, Korea, India, Thailand, and China. On my wife's recommendation, I started taking Hula lessons from a local Native Hawaiian bookstore called Na Mea Hawai'i. Through Hula and the wide range of Hawaiian literature, I discovered La'au Lapa'au, the traditional Native Hawaiian healer and healing practice. My passion of La'au Lapa'au took me on a great journey of both Hawaiiana and Native American history, culture, and knowledge.

Through this journey, I learned how Indigenous healing works and how to think about illness. When my wife's mother became diagnosed with cancer, I tried my best to help her through the things I learned, and perhaps my help worked in some sense, but in the quite opposite sense, she passed away. My passion to help people with sickness and cancer grew, and I felt so furious like others who know someone who passed away due to cancer, and more specifically, I felt furious because of the regret that there could have been a better way to treat my wife's mother's cancer. Was chemical therapy the best solution? Were the newest drugs available the best option or would something more traditional been better? Would taking no drugs at all been the best approach?

My wonder about cancer diminished when I started hearing about the concept that cancer is no longer a problem and people should not think about the word cancer and less in terms of a problem and more in terms of a treatment. This concept seemed to be addressing the public with the message that there were treatments for cancer, so you do not need to call it cancer anymore and you do you not need to talk about cancer either. This seemed to couple well with the information on cancer I was reading in Minnesota from a Native American perspective that cancer should not be talked or thought about because it can be caught by getting too involved.

When I started reading about the Indigenous research method, I came across a book on cancer that seemed to be just right for my involvement in healthcare as a data consultant and my last semester as a Masters of Public Health student. The book was called The Emperor of All Maladies: A Biography of Cancer, by Siddhartha Mukherjee. It was labeled as the Winner of the Pulitzer Prize and was named as a Top Ten Book of 2010 by "The New York Times," "O. The Oprah Magazine," and "Time," so I figured it was a light enough read to integrate me back into the world of cancer.

While reading this book, I decided to make the focus of my final master's paper, this paper, on cancer and cancer interventions, which would be analyzed through data from the University of Wisconsin Population Health Institute County Health Rankings and Roadmaps and from the Community Health Needs Assessment toolkits. The Emperor of All Maladies: A Biography of Cancer naturally draws the reader into the ambition to cure cancer through extravagant descriptions of dedicated individuals and overwhelming humanitarian cause, and I found it necessary to contribute towards the cure of cancer as well.

The one idea that stood out to me after finishing the book was that every physician considered cancer as evil, something like a black bile. However, the evil, black bile called cancer is described as a manner of treatment, and because there is not yet a complete cure for cancer, I thought there was something wrong with this understanding. Rather than repel the genetics of cancer, it should rather be embraced, specifically as an environmental adaptation in the evolutionary process. Humans should determine how their bodies evolve through their behavior. Yet it is not fair to those suffering from cancer to proclaim cancer as something to be embraced knowing humans cannot stop themselves from evolving; therefore, the understanding of cancer as something good needs to also be described through a manner of treatment. Fighting cancer with the most diabolical substances known to man may not be the best option. Something could have gone wrong when stumbling upon scientific advancements like x-rays and chemical therapy.

In deciding how to pursue a cure for cancer, I wanted to shy away from science as much as possible because the scientific method has yet to stop cancer from developing in the first place, so my choice of literature included three books on Charles Darwin, two course books on Public Health Law so as to remind myself of the boundaries of a public health intervention program, and a textbook called Health Psychology: Biopsychosocial Interactions to supplement biology and anatomy.

Shawn Wilson discussed in Research Is Ceremony: Indigenous Research Methods, that he wished he wrote more notes throughout his research and during conversations, so I took it upon myself to take notes during my research whenever an idea that sounded prosperous arose in my thoughts. The relationships between ideas that led me to my understanding of a cure for cancer from a public health standpoint was built upon ideas including those I noted down as follows:

My understanding is that the CHNA tools is that they focus on the micro rather than the macro level because the data is shown for specific counties and more specific populations as you zoom in. Would you consider it most important to think about more specific geographic populations and making connections or understand data across states or the country as a whole? (This was a question I posed during a County Health Rankings and Roadmaps presentation on CHNA)

Cancer is good in the sense of evolution. It should be embraced rather than scorned as a black bile.

Curing cancer is associated with money. A Program should increase value through money. People need to have more direction, directive, objective, and meaning in life through monetary value.

The octopus's eye is another connection in that the octopus sees like a human (even worse) but sees light and dark. The concept of seeing in light and dark may shine light onto a cure for cancer.

The parade is another possible connection to curing cancer. The American Dream Cancer.

It was recommended to stay away from too many metaphors in defining cancer. My metaphors will only be used on a personal note to formulate a cure for cancer through program planning.

My aim has to be to stop cancer through a remedy. Not find a cure, but stop it from beginning to develop. Not preventive. This is similar to tobacco prevention because not smoking decreases the chance of developing lung cancer, but people who don't smoke still get lung cancer.

I am not one to simply settle on an idea because of the necessity of producing results. While reading The Public Health Law Manual, by Frank P. Grad, searching for a cure for cancer, I came across my breakthrough. Grad wrote, "The court's disinclination to issue injunctions is reasonable in the light of the extraordinary nature of the remedy. An injunction is powerful medicine, for good or for evil." I immediately thought of the book Strong Medicine, by George C. Halvorson, the chairman and chief executive officer of Kaiser Permanente, who basically lays out the future of the healthcare system in his vision of the future. I happened to come across this book during an Ojibwa Powwow, so the term Strong Medicine had multiple connotations associated with both healing power and the healthcare system. I looked back at what injunctions were, and Grad wrote, "they were a common enforcement device in the control of air and water pollution." My thought was that if physicians or people approached air and water pollution as a cure for cancer with the same intensity and tenacity that they approached cancer through surgical procedures, heavy dosing of radioactive chemicals, and limitless genetic unraveling, then there might be some enormous improvements to the environment and to our health. There is clearly no evidence correlating air and water pollution to cancer through my idea, but this is not a scientific breakthrough, and it should therefore not be considered as such. Floyd Red Crow Westerman said in "Native American Prophecy", "Over 95% of our body is water. And, in order to stay healthy, you've got to drink good water. When the European first came here, Columbus, we could drink out of any river. If the Europeans had lived the Indian way when they came, we would still be drinking out of rivers, because Water is sacred. The Air is sacred."

There were still many questions to consider in determining how air and water pollution could be tackled through a public health intervention program. I was eating lunch at the Tin Fish Restaurant near Lake Calhoun in Minneapolis, Minnesota telling my parents about my research project, trying to explain how the Indigenous research methodology works and there was this big Indian looking guy, who from the front appeared to be a typical white guy, but from behind, you could see this super long braid, resembling the kind you see at a Powwow. I thought, I wonder what he would think about the macro vs. micro program planning effort for air and water pollution, which was a part of my original idea in utilizing data from either the micro (community level) or macro (national level). My father mentioned something about the horrific water pollution problem that has been ongoing now for some twenty odd years. Later that day, it dawned on me. One cannot possibly focus an air and water pollution initiative on one community because air and water is not restricted to that one area. It affects every community. The program must be directed on the macro level, or national level.

These breakthroughs of thought kept my mind preoccupied even while interacting with my family. I was playing with my son, laying on the carpet throwing a Styrofoam block up and down thinking about this void in my life that was left about concluding my writing career. Having written poetry and prose for 10 years, I really felt something missing. I know that I should fill this void with a life long work of controlling air and water pollution, but I just could not seem to grasp it or fit it into the void. Then it hit me. In my most recent paper on community health planning and evaluation, I included an advocacy project on sidewalk renovation and snow removal that was based on knowledge brokering. I decided then and there that I would build the air and water pollution program as an advocacy project, which could also be based on knowledge brokering. My son did not have much to say on the breakthrough because he was only 1 going on 2 years old, but if he could talk, I am sure he would have approved. I will let him read this paper later to show him what he might have missed.

I had my cure for cancer and I had my direction, but I still needed to know how to approach air and water pollution. My final breakthrough came from reading A Clear Mirror of Tibetan Medicinal Plants by Doctor Dawa. I was reading a book on Tibetan medicine in order to find a solution to the financially strained healthcare system. Based on today's healthcare system, hospitals and physician practices are turning in the direction of quality care, like Accountable Care Organizations, described by CMS as "groups of doctors, hospitals, and other health care providers, who come together voluntarily to give coordinated high quality care to their Medicare patients." To the best of my knowledge, the move towards quality care is similar to Tibetan medicine in that Tibetan medicine is renown for its long history of herbs and treatments approached from a scientific method. The financial incentive in America's healthcare system is in decline; however, through Tibetan medicine, the financial incentive can increase due to the high quality of this medicinal practice.

In the Introduction to this book, Men-Tsee-Khang of the Tibetan Medical & Astrological Institute wrote, "The unique system of Tibetan Medicine is not only broad and scientific but also has a long history and logic. The pollutant smoke of different chemicals which pollutes the nature and atmosphere affects the health of people to a great extent. Therefore, there is a growing interest and demand on the ancient authentic system of healing with the help of natural herbs. Taking this into consideration, and with the main aim to preserve and uplift the present traditional Tibetan Medicine, especially the herbs, and also to make easier for the people who are working on herbs, Doctor Dawa (sMan-Rampa), staff of Men-Tsee-Khang, paid much importance in bringing out the book on Tibetan Medicinal Herbs." It would make much sense to incorporate the future of healthcare into a community health program. The focus of a public health intervention would be to determine how the balance of the environment affects cancer. My goal is to obtain data through the County Health Rankings and Roadmaps and the Community Health Needs Assessment toolkits and compare to my findings on the environment including surrounding plants and nature. As a long-term outcome, I would like to understand the balance of plants and determine how to implement changes through advocacy to reach that balance so cancer can be cured.

Bibliography
Appleman, P. (ed). 2001. Darwin (3rd ed.). New York, NY: W. W. Norton & Company, Inc.
Community Health Needs Assessment (CHNA) toolkit (http://CHNA.org/)
County Health Rankings and Roadmap (http://www.countyhealthrankings.org/)
Darwin, C. 1985. The Origin of Species. New York, NY: Penguin Books.
Friis, R. 2012. Essentials of Environmental Health (2nd ed.). Sudbury, MA: Jones & Bartlett Learning, LLC.
Gribbin, J. and M. Gribbin. 1997. Darwin in 90 Minutes. London, England: Constable and Company Limited.
Sarafino, E. and T. Smith. 2011. Health Psychology (7th ed.). John Wiley & Sons Inc.
Wing, K., W. Mariner, G. Annas, and D. Strouse. 2007. Public Health Law. Newark, NJ: Matthew Bender & Company, Inc.

References

CMS. Accountable Care Organizations. Retrived June 15, 2013.
http://www.cms.gov/Medicare/Medicare-Fee-for-Service-Payment/ACO/index.html?redirect=%2Faco%2F

Dawa, D. 1999. A Clear Mirror of Tibetan Medicinal Plants. Rome, Italy: Tiet Domani.

Grad, F. 2005. The Public Health Law Manual (3rd ed.). Washington, DC: American Public Health Association.

Mukherjee, S. 2010. The Emperor of All Maladies: A Biography of Cancer. New York, NY: Scribner.

Westerman, Floyd Red Crow. Native American Prophecy. Retrieved June 17, 2013. http://astructureforspirit.com/2011/12/09/native-american-prophecy/

Wilson, S. 2008. Research Is Ceremony: Indigenous Research Methods. Winnipeg, Manitoba: Fernwood Publishing.

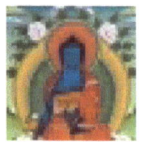

America's Healthcare Plan: A Strategy for Achieving Quality Care

July 12

The National Quality Strategy of the Affordable Care Act established three aims including:
1. Better Care
2. Healthy People/Healthy Communities
3. Affordable Care
My health plan is addressing numbers 1 and 3. My work on renewable fuel is addressing 2, but more importantly, my work on finding a cure for cancer through air and water pollution controls is valuable to the second initiative, so I am posting my paper titled Finding a Cure for Cancer Utilizing the Indigenous Research Method here.

Like · · Share

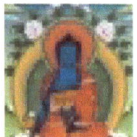

America's Healthcare Plan: A Strategy for Achieving Quality Care

July 12

To gain a complete understanding of all of America's cultures, a Gandhian approach should be taken by traveling around America, American Territories, and Tribal Nations so as to see and experience all the different cultures attributing to a health care plan.

1Like · · Share

[America's Healthcare Plan: A Strategy for Achieving Quality Care](#)

I will have to do it from my home, like the armchair anthropologist, because I do not have the finances to fund such an expedition at this time.

July 12 at 10:40am · Like

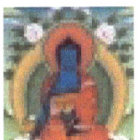

America's Healthcare Plan: A Strategy for Achieving Quality Care

July 12

I will substitute Healthcare System with culture and substitute Health Plan with happiness and substitute Medical Care with Quality-Care, which looks like the following:
Culture
|
Happiness
|
Quality-Care

Like · · Share

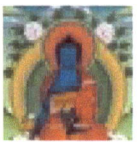

America's Healthcare Plan: A Strategy for Achieving Quality Care

July 12

Through timing there is happiness. Why? Because of freedom. America is the country of the land of the free and the people have the right to pursuit happiness. A health plan is meant to cater to this correlation.

1Like · · Share

America's Healthcare Plan: A Strategy for Achieving Quality Care

What is the ultimate point of timing, strategy, and tolerance? To succeed. To achieve. To live. The most important outcome of timing: happiness, is the outcome of all these points.

July 12 at 8:13am · Like

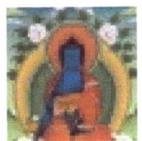

[America's Healthcare Plan: A Strategy for Achieving Quality Care](#)

[July 11](#)

Writing comments on facebook is much easier than writing a paper or a book. I have decided to stop actually writing a paper on America's Healthcare Plan and just keep writing my thoughts and conclusions as status updates. I am not sure if I will copy and paste them over to a book later or how that would work.

[1Like](#) · · [Share](#)

[America's Healthcare Plan: A Strategy for Achieving Quality Care](#)

I just tried making a pdf and a word document and it seems like it would work well, but I will definitely need to format it correctly.

[July 11 at 10:04pm](#) · [Like](#)

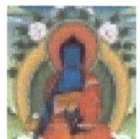

[America's Healthcare Plan: A Strategy for Achieving Quality Care](#)

[July 11](#)

I would like to start numbering different types of culture I see, but, like trying to remember a dream after waking, I just seem to forget when I get home. So, for now, my numbers will be blank.

1.
2.
3.
4.
5.

[Like](#) · · [Share](#)

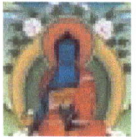

[America's Healthcare Plan: A Strategy for Achieving Quality Care](#)

[July 11](#)

I will also be exploring tolerance, which I have not defined or understood the connotation of, but similar to strategy, tolerance emerges through timing or it is an output of timing.

[Like](#) · · [Share](#)

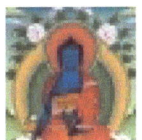

America's Healthcare Plan: A Strategy for Achieving Quality Care

July 11

Defining culture is enjoyable by gazing out into society in my daily life. The challenge is understanding culture in broader terms by including all cultures a healthcare plan would cover including American Territories and Tribal Nations not to mention all different classes and subcultures of people.

1Like · · Share

America's Healthcare Plan: A Strategy for Achieving Quality Care

The good part is that there is no need to read textbooks and spend countless hours in the library just to identify culture. Then, after culture is identified, or rather in the identification of culture, the healthcare strategy will emerge.

July 11 at 9:46pm · Like

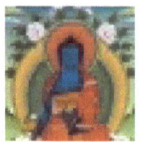

America's Healthcare Plan: A Strategy for Achieving Quality Care

July 11

The healthcare system is a complex, nontransparent, unstructured organization of various entities, laws, and economics. To articulate the organization of a healthcare system, it is most clear to lay out the hierarchy of medicine:

Healthcare system
|
Health Plan
|
Medical Care

5Like · · Share

America's Healthcare Plan: A Strategy for Achieving Quality Care

Despite complex systems, simplicity is possible, and simplicity is the most transparent.

July 11 at 5:02pm · Like

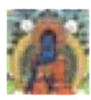

America's Healthcare Plan: A Strategy for Achieving Quality Care

The key then of a health system is to simplify complex organizations.

July 11 at 5:02pm · Like

America's Healthcare Plan: A Strategy for Achieving Quality Care

That being said, Tibetan's systems of organization are incredibly complex and intricate, but they are still transparent. How is that possible?

July 11 at 5:03pm · Like

America's Healthcare Plan: A Strategy for Achieving Quality Care

I know why.... Because the systems are functions of culture. Or in other words, the systems of organization are outcomes and/or they are related to the culture.

July 11 at 5:05pm · Like

America's Healthcare Plan: A Strategy for Achieving Quality Care

The systems are the culture therefore, if complex systems are necessary for operations, then they should be a part of the culture.

July 11 at 5:06pm · Like

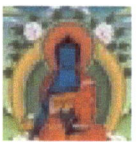

America's Healthcare Plan: A Strategy for Achieving Quality Care

July 11

Time, time, time, time time... How does time translate into a social function of life? I know it is possible through mathematics, but I will figure it out through program planning.

3Like · · Share

America's Healthcare Plan: A Strategy for Achieving Quality Care

If considered backwards, then strategy is an outcome of time.

July 11 at 4:47pm · Like

America's Healthcare Plan: A Strategy for Achieving Quality Care

Strategy is a much easier concept to grasp, but it does not fully explain how timing improves a health plan. Timing leads to much more than strategy.

July 11 at 4:49pm · Like

America's Healthcare Plan: A Strategy for Achieving Quality Care

Timing is the basis of America's health plan.
or
Timing is America's health plan.
or
Timing = America's health plan

July 11 at 4:55pm · Like

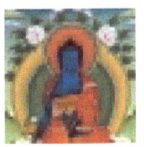

America's Healthcare Plan: A Strategy for Achieving Quality Care

July 11

When looking out at the healthcare plans of America and the healthcare system with fresh eyes, what do you see? At first glance, I see emptiness. No existence whatsoever. This means that there are limitless possibilities to implement an effective plan. People exist and socioeconomic factors affect people. A healthcare plan should cater to the needs of the people.

Like · · Share

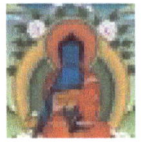

America's Healthcare Plan: A Strategy for Achieving Quality Care shared a link.

July 11

I guess my initiative is also a bit of an advocacy project. I would like to think of wind power knowledge broker, Philip Warburg, who has demonstrated advocacy for renewable-energy with a focus on wind power and the contributions it can make to America's energy future. Philip Warburg articulates why fossil fuels and nuclear power are not good long-term options for US energy; why wind power is an ideal alternative; and what the US will have to do to build its wind-power capacity to fulfill 20% of the nation's energy needs by 2030.

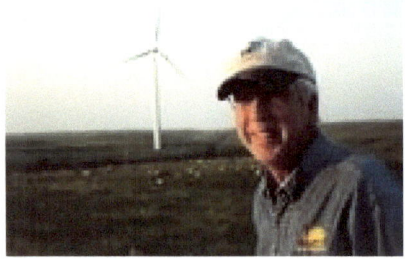

Official Website - Author of Harvest the Wind - Philip Warburg

philipwarburg.com

Official website for Philip Warburg, author of Harvest the Wind: America's Journey to Jobs, Energy Independence, and Climate Stability - Wind Power and Alternative Energy

3Like · · Share

[America's Healthcare Plan: A Strategy for Achieving Quality Care](#)

Following suit with Warburg's work on wind power, I am also working on a different community program planning project that will articulate why gasoline is not a good long-term option for US automobile fuel; why ethanol is an ideal alternative; and what the US will have to do to implement ethanol as an alternative fuel.

July 11 at 12:17pm · Like

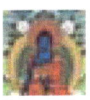

[America's Healthcare Plan: A Strategy for Achieving Quality Care](#)

Health and air pollution are most definitely linked. I will be using data from County Health Rankings and Roadmaps on daily fine particulate matter including the average daily measure of fine particulate matter in micrograms per cubic meter (PM2.5) in a county and on health-related quality of life to compare effects of fuel consumption and ethanol fuel initiatives to be demonstrated on a national level, then develop an intervention program plan.

July 11 at 12:24pm · Like

[America's Healthcare Plan: A Strategy for Achieving Quality Care](#)

The major question regarding a healthcare plan and quality-care, is how far should the plan and treatment be taken? Should environmental factors be included? Population-based medicine is a key component of preventive medicine.

July 11 at 12:26pm · Like

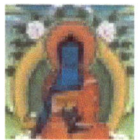

[America's Healthcare Plan: A Strategy for Achieving Quality Care](#)

[July 11](#)

I am still formulating my concept of timing as a key component of a healthcare plan. In my opinion, the basis of America's success is timing. Through timing, strategy can be implemented and relationships can be built. In the age of massive amounts of data, information, and multitude of organizational hierarchies, relationships are all that we can hold onto.

[Like](#) · · [Share](#)

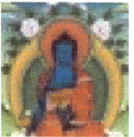

[America's Healthcare Plan: A Strategy for Achieving Quality Care](#)

[July 11](#)

The purpose of my health plan is to make it financially possible to delivery high-quality healthcare. All I hear as a member of the general public is how bad the economy is and how economically strapped the healthcare system is. I am not completely sure if this is the case, but I do know from being the healthcare industry for 7 years and working towards a Doctorate in Public Health, that the current system is unsustainable unless interventions are put in place.

[2Like](#) · · [Share](#)

[America's Healthcare Plan: A Strategy for Achieving Quality Care](#)

The one argument against the fact that the current healthcare system is unsustainable, is that there exists a natural curve that is bringing balance to the economics of the healthcare system. Specifically, this is the sense that insurance companies are putting more financial responsibility onto the patient with higher deductibles and hospitals are attempting to make their operations more efficient.

July 11 at 11:41am · Like

[America's Healthcare Plan: A Strategy for Achieving Quality Care](#)

This natural curve, however, is in part dependent on a the successful implementation of high-quality medical care through organizations like Accountable Care Organizations. There are very few incentives of quality-care to the physicians and to the hospitals and that is where Tibetan Medicine contributes because of the high-quality efficient standard of Tibetan Medicine.

July 11 at 11:43am · Like

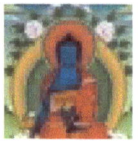

America's Healthcare Plan: A Strategy for Achieving Quality Care

July 11

Despite the intricate and complex organization of Tibetan social, political, and religious entities, their structure is transparent. America's healthcare system may be as dynamic and complex as the organization in Tibet; however, it is not transparent and easy to follow. The structure and organization of America's healthcare system is the product of laws, business entities like insurance companies, hospitals, and physician practices, and the government, which are only to mention a few of them. Due to the large amount of data and literature on America's healthcare system, it is a valuable tool to identify concepts based on relationships between ideas to gain a full understanding of the current healthcare system, upon which a well-rounded perspective can be applied to construct an ideal health plan.

Like · · Share

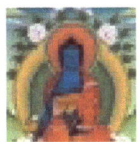

America's Healthcare Plan: A Strategy for Achieving Quality Care

July 11

To understand Tibetan medicine, the history of Tibet is a good place to start. The history of Tibet is very long due to the literature that has been recorded internally and externally through interactions with China and surrounding countries as well as with Russia and Europe. The depth and breadth of the books on Tibetan history requires great knowledge to fully comprehend. Due to the vast amount of material on the subject and complexity of interpreting historical documents, retelling the history or even summarizing the history would detract from the purpose to describe how Tibetan medicine can help improve America's healthcare system.

4Like · · Share

America's Healthcare Plan: A Strategy for Achieving Quality Care

When deciding how to proceed in transmitting the value and importance of Tibetan history, it is beneficial to focus on the relationships between ideas, whether they are relationships within the historical context or in the contemporary context. There are three main concepts that emerged through relationships realized in my readings of Tibetan history that will provide enough contextual understanding of the relationship between Tibetan history and Tibetan medicine and how it is applied to America's healthcare system.

July 11 at 12:57am · Like

[America's Healthcare Plan: A Strategy for Achieving Quality Care](#)

The first concept is that Tibetan history reveals Tibet's extravagant and complex governmental, religious, and social structures. The composition of each entity has been organized to an immense degree. This is important because it shines light on the limitations and lack of organization of our current healthcare system.

July 11 at 1:03am · Edited · Like

[America's Healthcare Plan: A Strategy for Achieving Quality Care](#)

The second concept is that prior to Buddhism, Tibet was a nation immersed in commerce and political conflict. This is important because it introduces an important perspective to the contemporary, external view of Tibet, which is that of a compassionate, Buddhist people. This might seem like an obvious historical fact, yet it is actually very difficult to fully acknowledge that Tibet existed as a completely different organized state because of the intricate, profound, and mysterious image of modern Tibet. To fully acknowledge Tibet's existence as a major political and economic entity prior to Buddhism is to appreciate Tibet's knowledge and experiences.

July 11 at 12:57am · Like

[America's Healthcare Plan: A Strategy for Achieving Quality Care](#)

The third concept is that medicine is not discussed in great detail in history books despite that the traditional Tibetan medical system is one of the Five Major Studies of Tibet with an equally long history, and that the primary contemporary context of Tibetan medicine is a body of knowledge constructed through the gathering of Tibetan historical medical knowledge similar to how a bee gathers pollen from flowers. This is important in that without knowing everything about Tibetan medicine, the value of Tibetan medicine can be reproduced; therefore, it is not necessary to study the body of knowledge of Tibetan medicine. It can be applied immediately to America's healthcare system.

[July 11 at 12:58am](#) · [Like](#)

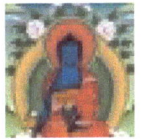

[America's Healthcare Plan: A Strategy for Achieving Quality Care](#)

[July 10](#)

High quality medicine must be based on a high quality healthcare system, which is why I am focusing on the health plan itself prior to explaining Tibetan medicine and how Tibetan medicine will help shape quality-care treatments in America.

[2Like](#) · · [Share](#)

America's Healthcare Plan: A Strategy for Achieving Quality Care

This concept is based on research of Tibetan Medicine. There is actually not so much literature on Tibetan Medicine, or at least at first glance. When searching for Tibetan Medicine at St. Thomas University Library, I was directed to the section on Tibet. All the literature on Tibet was on history and culture. I made a connection that the foundations of history are important to Tibet, therefore the foundations of a healthcare system are important in medicine.

July 10 at 2:54pm · Like

America's Healthcare Plan: A Strategy for Achieving Quality Care

I did make it to the medical section of the library and found more on Ayurveda then Tibetan Medicine; however, I am utilizing Ayurveda moreso as a component to Native American Shamanism than as a quality-care medical treatment.

July 10 at 2:56pm · Like

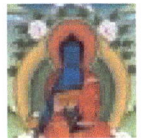

[America's Healthcare Plan: A Strategy for Achieving Quality Care](#)

[July 9](#)

Who is to be covered by America's Health Plan? How are America's territories treated? How are tribal nations treated?

[Like](#) · · [Share](#)

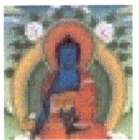

[America's Healthcare Plan: A Strategy for Achieving Quality Care](#) changed their [cover photo](#).

[July 9](#)

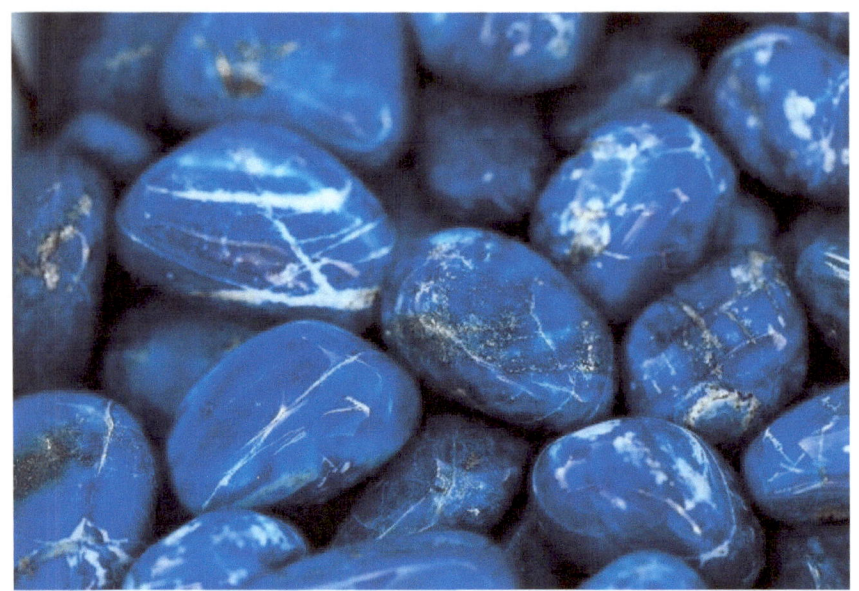

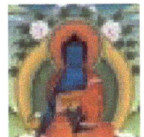

[America's Healthcare Plan: A Strategy for Achieving Quality Care](#)

[July 9](#)

The key to America's healthcare plan is timing.

[1Like](#) · · [Share](#)

[America's Healthcare Plan: A Strategy for Achieving Quality Care](#)

I will go into more detail later.

[July 10 at 2:52pm](#) · [Like](#)

Joined Facebook

July 8

www.ingramcontent.com/pod-product-compliance
Lightning Source LLC
Chambersburg PA
CBHW050826290526
45792CB00001B/273